How Billy (the Kidney) Earned His Name

A Kidney Transplant Book for Kids

Stephanie Peters, Psy.D., LP

Kendra Read, Ph.D.

DEDICATION

To all the kids and kidneys.

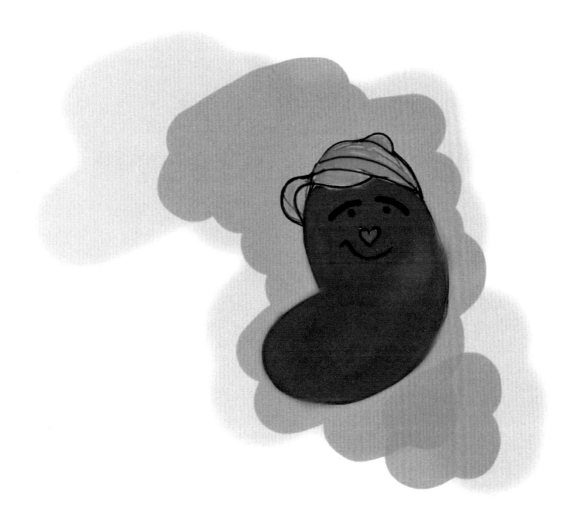

My name is Billy (the Kidney)—but that wasn't always my name.

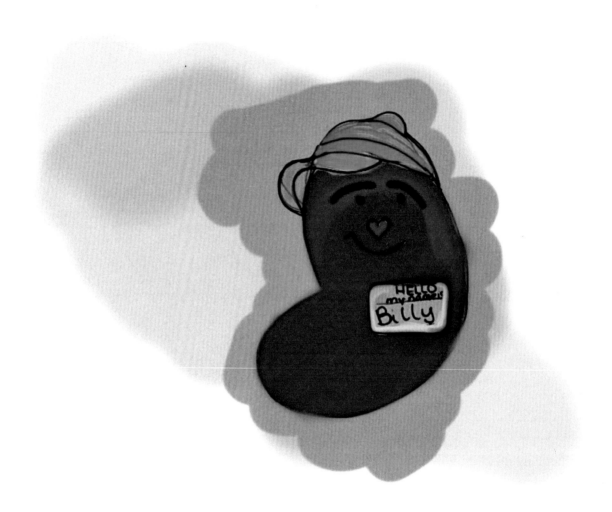

Although I don't remember what I used to be called, I do remember the
wonderful day I got the name Billy (the Kidney). It was the same day I had
my great big adventure!

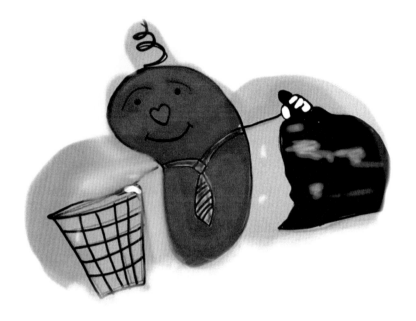

Before that day, most of my days were the same. I worked hard keeping The Body's blood clean from trash, making trash into urine (a fancy name for "pee"), and releasing chemicals into The Body to keep it healthy and strong.

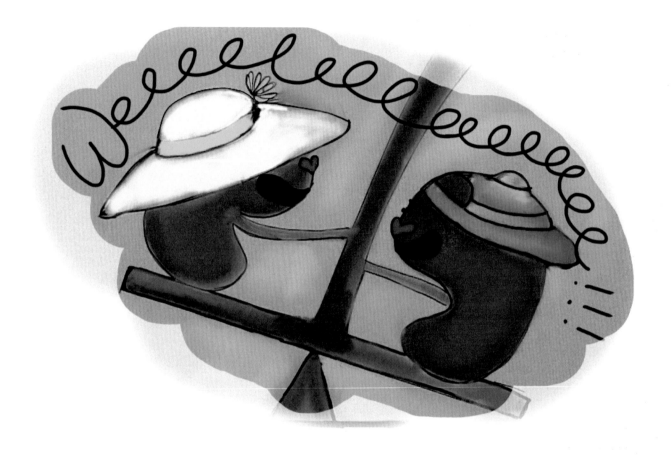

There's always a lot of work to be done by us kidneys. In fact, there is so much to be done that we kidneys usually work in pairs. Doctors only split up a good kidney team if there is an important reason.

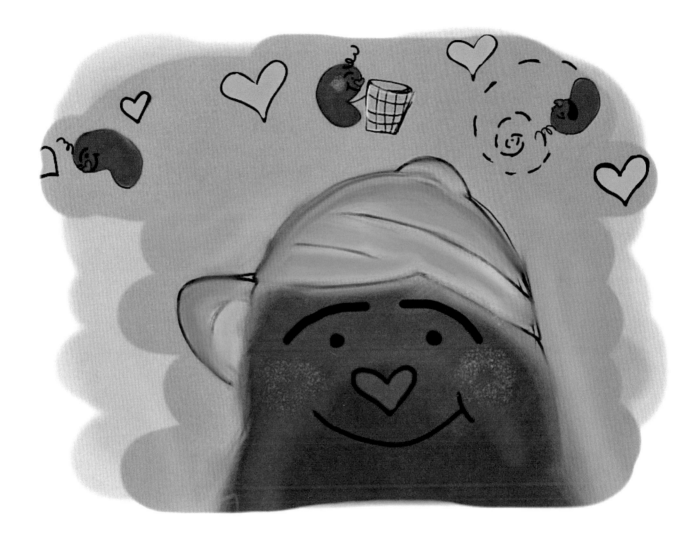

There are some nice perks to working in The Body: it's always warm and cozy. Plus, who can complain about a steady job? I'm often so busy with work, I forget what day it is. But I'll always remember the day I had my great big adventure!

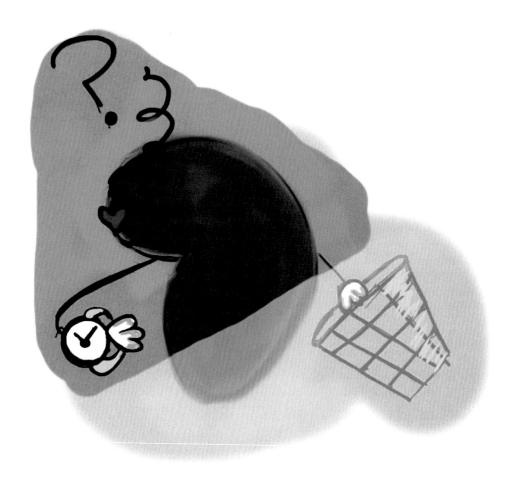

The day of my great big adventure started like any other day. I was focused on getting the morning trash filtering out of the way, but there wasn't much work.

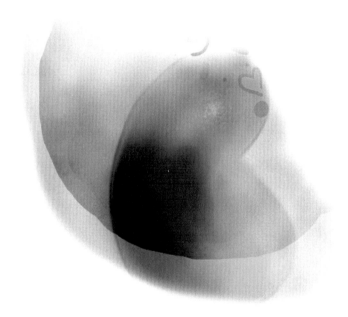

Suddenly, I saw a light! I was astonished by its brightness and beauty; it was the first time I had ever seen light. I heard a strong and in-charge voice say:

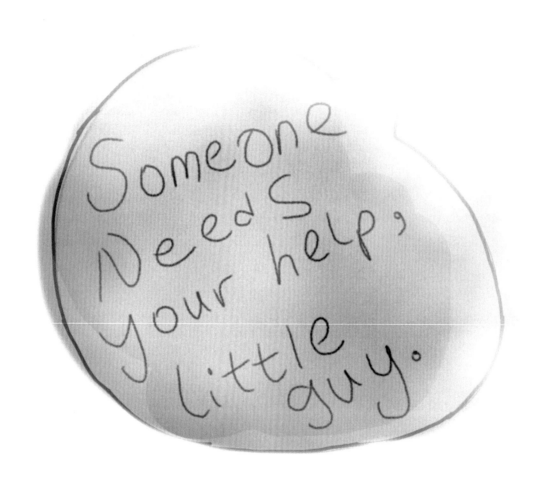

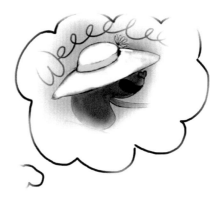

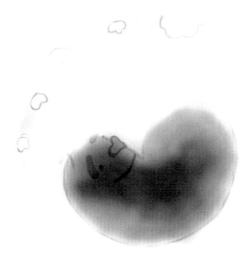

It was then that I realized: I was OUT OF THE BODY. What a strange out-of-Body experience. I trusted my kidney partner to keep up the great work we had been doing.

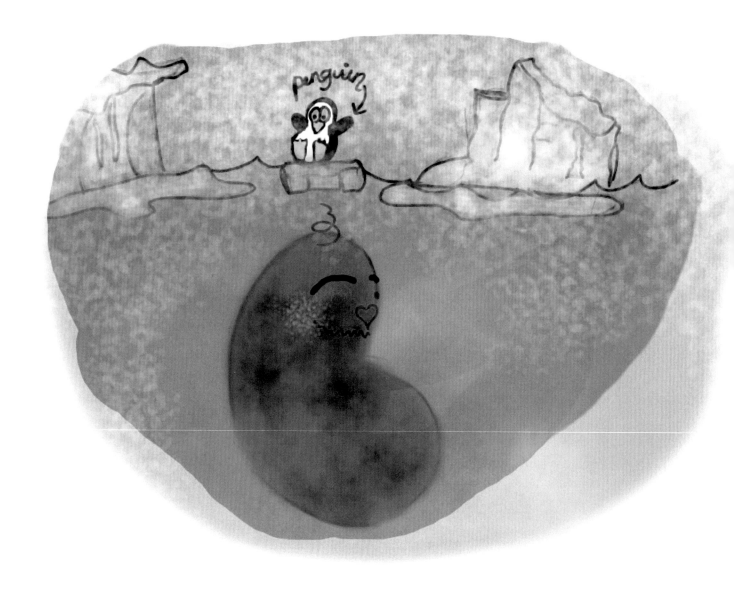

Then, I felt cold like I was plunged in an icy slush. I remember when The Body was learning about the arctic. I bet it was at least that cold!

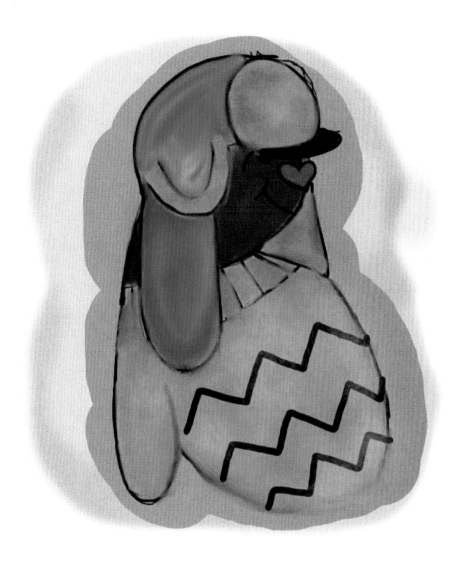

It would have been nice if someone had sent me a memo—I could have brought my hat and mitten.

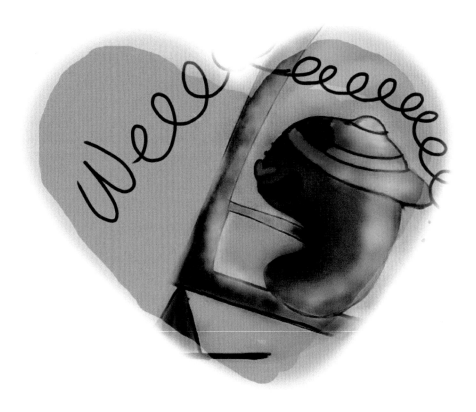

After feeling cold (and curious about what would happen next) I was placed in a NEW BODY! What a great big adventure!

There was a lot of work to do in the New Body so I got started right away.

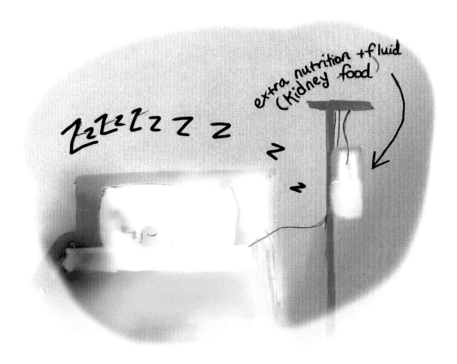

I overheard that the New Body needed to stay in the hospital for a little while.
The doctors wanted to be close while I got used to working in a new place.

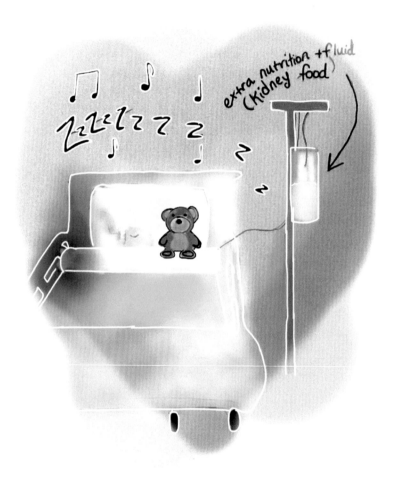

Even though it was normal for the New Body to feel uncomfortable, the doctors worked hard to make her as comfy as possible.

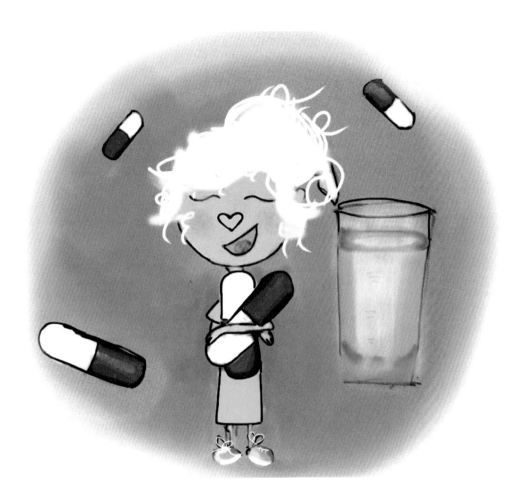

Once I entered the New Body, I had to tango with her new-to-me immune system. The immune system protects the bodies from unwanted visitors. To stop her immune system from kicking me out, she took some medications that marked me as a safe visitor. Every time the New Body took her medications, it was like she was saying I could stay and work!

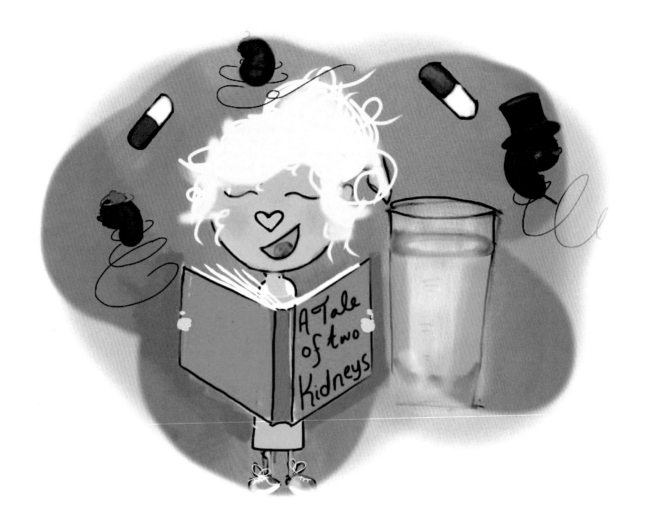

As hard as I was working to get everything up and running, the New Body was learning all about little old me! She was studying about how to take all of her medications, follow a new diet, drink the right amount of water, and get plenty of rest.

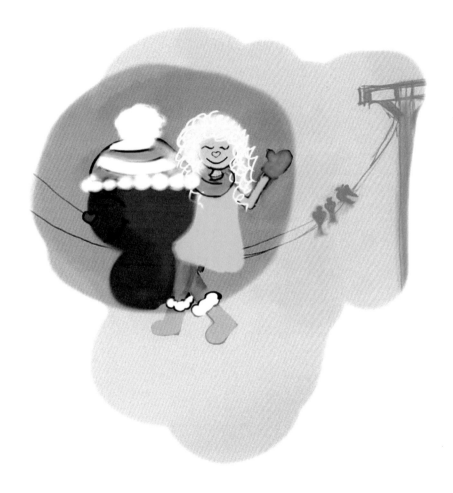

Pretty soon, we were BFFs. I felt grateful that we were always together (just like peas and carrots, or birds on telephone wires) working to keep her healthy and strong.

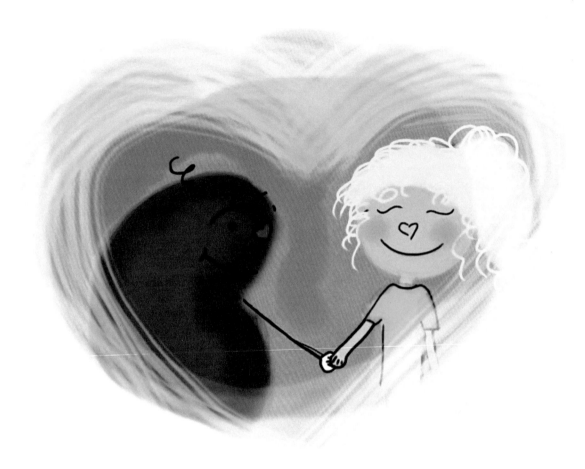

As the New Body and I worked together, I overheard her say "Thank you Billy (the Kidney) for everything you do for me." What an amazingly cool name and cool New Body! I've been telling everyone to call me "Billy" ever since.

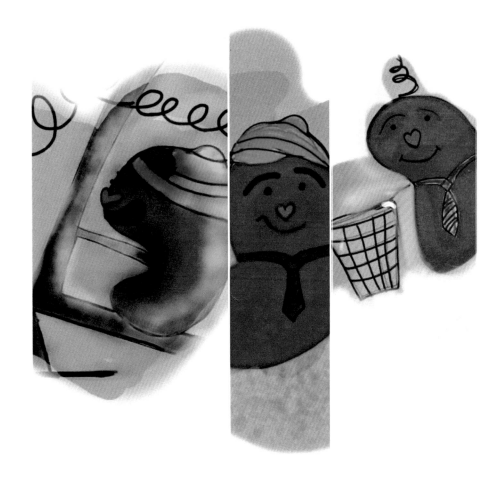

Soon enough, I was back to my old routine, turning trash into urine (among other things) and keeping the New Body's fluids in tip-top shape. I sometimes even forget that I ever had a great big adventure…

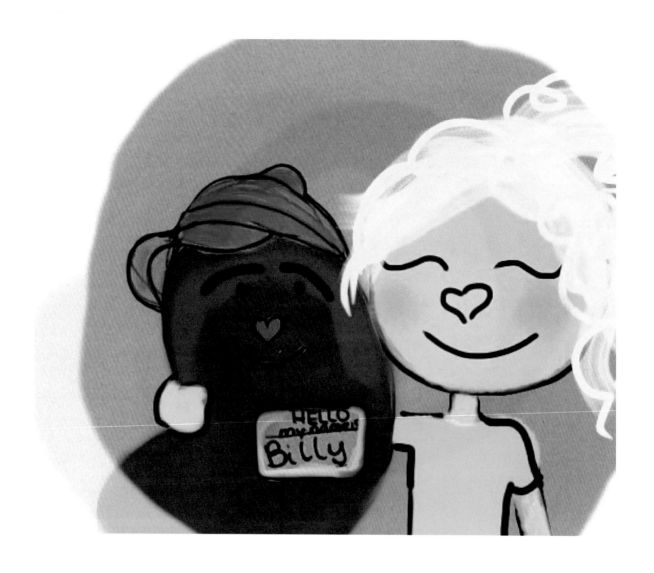

…but then I remember my awesome name and the special human I'm working hard for every day.

What is your kidney's name?

_____

What makes your kidney happy?

_____

_____

What is its favorite music?

_____

_____

How are you keeping your kidney protected in its new body?

_____

_____

_____

_____

_____

Write your own kidney story:

Draw a picture of your new kidney:

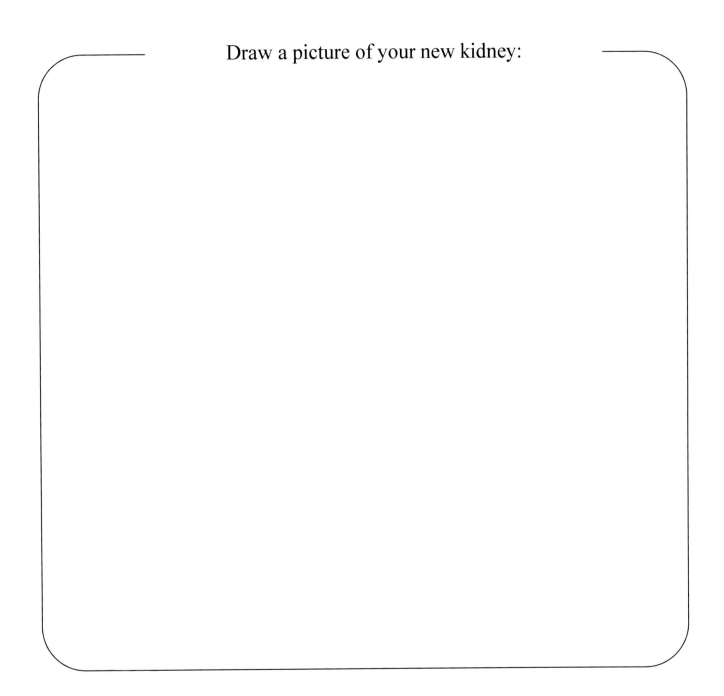

Draw a picture of your new kidney wearing his favorite hat:

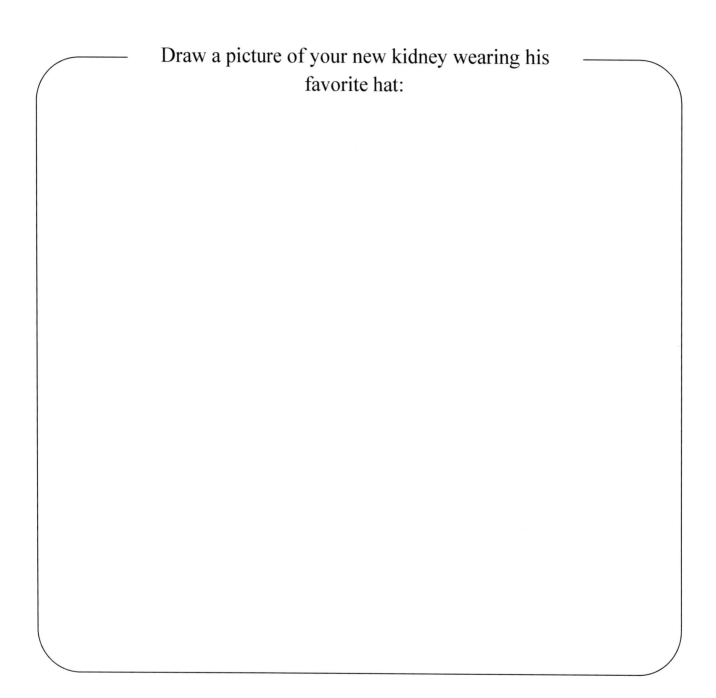

Here is a **chart** to help you learn the medications you need to keep your kidney working hard!

Name of medication:	Draw a picture of it!	At what time should I take this?	How much should I take?	What makes this medication important?

Hint: Some kids make a new chart every time their medications change to help them remember what they need to help their kidney.

Here is a **schedule** to help you keep track of the days and times you are remembering to take your medications!

Date:	Medication Name:	How much?	Time 1:	Time 2:	Time 3:

Hint: Some kids set alarms on their cell phones to help them remember when they need to take their medication.

Parent Hint: Some parents keep their own tracking sheet and give small rewards when possible every time their child takes his/her medication.

Here is a **schedule** to help you remember to drink the fluid you need to keep your body healthy!

Date:	Amount of fluid I need:	Time 1: Did I reach my goal?	Time 2: Did I reach my goal?	Time 3: Did I reach my goal?	Time 4: Did I reach my goal?

Hint: Instead of drinking fluid all at once, some kids figure out how much they need to drink hour by hour to make their goal.

Parent Hint: Some parents keep their own tracking sheet and give small rewards when their child drinks his/her fluid.

Make a list of people who you can call if you have any questions—or if you notice you are having a hard time taking your medications on time:

1. _____

2. _____

3. _____

4. _____

5. _____

6. _____

Hint: Your doctors and nurses could go on this list.

About the Authors

Dr. Stephanie Peters is a licensed clinical psychologist and health care consultant who has specialized training in treating children and families impacted by acute and chronic medical conditions. She worked with children in all stages of the kidney transplant process during her predoctoral internship at Jackson Memorial Hospital and postdoctoral fellowship at Stanford University School of Medicine. She currently lives in Minneapolis, Minnesota.

Dr. Kendra Read is a licensed clinical psychologist, currently working as the Director of Anxiety Programs at Seattle Children's Hospital and an acting assistant professor at the University of Washington School of Medicine. She completed her doctorate at Temple University, including her pediatric psychology internship at Nemours/A.I duPont Hospital for Children in Wilmington, Delaware and her postdoctoral fellowship at Stanford University School of Medicine. She currently lives in Seattle, Washington.

Made in the USA
Lexington, KY
12 July 2018